CKD STAGE 4

DIET

COOKBOOK

FOR SENIORS

The Ultimate Guide with 20 Delicious & Easy Recipes for Managing Chronic Kidney Disease in Your Golden Years

Patricia Camire

CHECK OTHER BOOKS BY AUTHOR:

TABLE OF CONTENT

INTRODUCTION

In the wonderful story of Emily, a vivacious senior navigating life with CKD Stage 4, the CKD Stage 4 Diet Cookbook served as a guiding light.

Faced with dietary restrictions, Emily uncovered a treasure mine of 20 tasty and simple dishes adapted to her unique requirements.

Each page seemed like a gourmet expedition, exposing her to kidney-friendly products and basic cooking skills.

Emily underwent a miraculous turnaround after embracing the cookbook's lessons. Her meals were a symphony of flavors that balanced nutrition and taste.

With increased energy, she confidently strolled the shopping aisles, selecting items that not only improved her kidney health but also pleased her taste senses.

The cookbook's useful advice and time-saving methods transformed dinner preparation into a joyful ritual. Emily discovered not just nourishment but also a fresh feeling of strength on her culinary adventure, with each meal serving as a celebration of health and vigor.

The CKD Stage 4 Diet Cookbook became more than just a collection of dishes; it became Emily's trusty companion on her journey to health.

CHAPTER ONE

UNDERSTANDING CKD STAGE 4 AND NUTRITION

As we begin our journey to comprehend Chronic Kidney Disease (CKD) Stage 4 and the importance of diet in treating this illness, it is critical that we approach this chapter with clarity and simplicity, bearing in mind our valued elders' special requirements.

Introduction to Chronic Kidney Disease (CKD), Stage 4

Chronic Kidney Disease is a prevalent health condition, particularly among the elderly. In this chapter, we will look at the characteristics of CKD Stage 4, which is an important stage in the evolution of renal disease.

Imagine your kidneys as industrious filters that clean your blood, eliminating waste and extra fluids to maintain your body in balance.

With CKD Stage 4, these filters are substantially degraded, reducing their capacity to function properly.

Understanding the stage of your kidney illness is critical for managing your health properly.

The Role of Nutrition in CKD Stage 4 Management

Now let's get to the heart of the matter: how diet may be a great ally in controlling CKD Stage 4. What you eat is important for maintaining kidney function and general health.

Key Nutrients:

- **Low-phosphorus foods**: Because phosphorus can build in the blood with renal disease, eating low-phosphorus meals such as fresh fruits, vegetables, and lean meats is critical.

- **Reduced sodium intake**: Limiting salt consumption helps manage blood pressure and fluid balance, reducing the strain on your kidneys.

- **Balanced protein consumption**: Maintaining a healthy protein intake is critical. Choose high-quality foods such as chicken, fish, and eggs, but be aware of quantity sizes.

CKD-Friendly Ingredients and Cooking Methods

Navigating the shopping aisles with CKD Stage 4 requires selecting items that are both appetizing and kidney-friendly.

Kidney-Friendly Ingredients:

- **Fresh fruits and vegetables**: Choose a rainbow of hues to acquire a range of nutrients.

- **Whole grains**: Brown rice, quinoa, and whole wheat pasta all be nutritious options.

- **Lean proteins**: Fish, skinless poultry, and eggs are great protein sources with low phosphorus levels.

Cooking techniques include grilling and baking, which improve tastes without using excessive oil or salt.

- Herb and spice infusion: Experimenting with herbs and spices enhances the flavor of your recipes while being healthy.

Lifestyle Changes for CKD Stage 4

Beyond the kitchen, lifestyle changes can have a huge influence on your CKD Stage 4 journey.

Ensure proper hydration by drinking enough water. Staying hydrated improves kidney function. Keep track of your fluid intake to stay in balance.

Exercise:

- **Gentle physical activity**: Light workouts such as walking or tai chi might improve general well-being.

- **Stress management** involves mindfulness techniques. Use relaxation techniques like deep breathing or meditation to reduce tension.

Meal Planning Tips and Time-Saving Strategies

Now, let's make dinner preparation more practical and pleasurable.

Meal Planning:

- **Weekly Planning**: Outline your weekly meals to achieve a balanced and diverse diet.

- **Cook in bulk and Refrigerate for later use**. - Use pre-cut veggies to save time and effort.

- **One-pot wonders**: Simplify your culinary routine with one-pot recipes that are simple to make and clean up.

Remember, the objective is to make your meals both healthy and pleasurable while meeting your dietary requirements in CKD Stage 4.

In this Chapter, we've created the framework for understanding CKD Stage 4 by emphasizing the significance of diet, researching kidney-friendly substances, and making lifestyle changes.

As we go on to Chapter 2, prepare to embark on a culinary adventure with 20 delicious and easy CKD-friendly recipes designed exclusively for our loving elders.

Your health is our first priority, and we're here for you every step of the way.

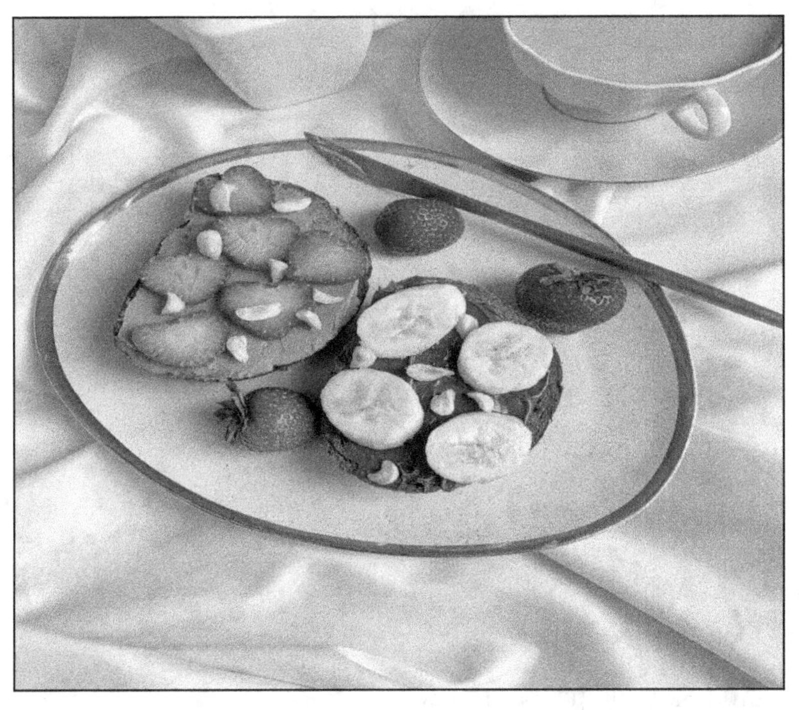

CHAPTER TWO

DELICIOUS CKD STAGE 4 DIET RECIPES

1. Grilled Lemon Herb Chicken

Ingredients:

- 4 boneless, skinless chicken breasts

- 2 tablespoons of olive oil

- 2 tablespoons of fresh lemon juice

- 1 teaspoon of dry oregano

- One teaspoon of dried thyme

- Add Salt and pepper to taste

Preparation:

1. Combine olive oil, lemon juice, oregano, thyme, salt, and pepper to make a marinade.

2. Put the chicken breasts in a resealable plastic bag and pour the marinade over them. Seal the bag and freeze for minimum of 30 minutes.

3. Preheat the grill to medium-high.

4. Grill the chicken for 6-8 minutes per side, or until well done.

5. Serve alongside steamed veggies or a fresh salad.

Prep Time: 40 minutes (including marination)

Servings: 4

2. Quinoa and Vegetable Stir-Fry

Ingredients:

- 1 cup quinoa, washed

- 2 cups of water

- 1 tablespoon of olive oil

- 1 sliced onion,

- 2 julienned carrots,

- 1 sliced bell pepper,

- 1 cup of trimmed snap peas,

- 2 tablespoons of low-sodium soy sauce

- One teaspoon of grated ginger

Preparation:

1. In a saucepan, mix quinoa and water. Bring to a boil, then decrease heat, cover, and simmer for 15-20 minutes, or until the quinoa is done.

2. In a large pan, increase the olive oil temperature over medium-high heat.

3. Combine the onion, carrots, bell pepper, and snap peas. Stir-fry the veggies for 5-7 minutes, or until soft and crisp.

4. Add the cooked quinoa to the skillet.

5. In a small bowl, combine the soy sauce and grated ginger. Toss the quinoa and veggies together.

6. Serve hot.

Prep Time: 30 minutes

Servings: 4

3. Berry and Greek Yogurt Parfait

Ingredients:

- Two cups of Greek yogurt

- 1 cup of mixed berries such as strawberries, blueberries, and raspberries

- 2 tablespoons of honey

- 1/4 cup of chopped nuts such as almonds or walnuts

Preparation:

1. Layer Greek yogurt, mixed berries, and chopped almonds in serving glasses.

2. Drizzle the honey over each parfait.

3. Repeat the layers until the glass is full.

4. Refrigerate for at least 30 minutes before serving.

Prep Time: 10 minutes

Servings: 2

4. Baked Salmon with Lemon-Dill Sauce

Ingredients:

- 4 salmon fillets

- 1 tablespoon of olive oil

- 1 sliced lemon,

- 2 tablespoons of chopped fresh dill,

- Add Salt and pepper to taste

Preparation:

1. Preheat oven to 375°F (190°C).

2. Arrange salmon fillets on a baking pan.

3. Drizzle olive oil over the fish, then season with salt and pepper.

4. Garnish each fillet with lemon slices and fresh dill.

5. Bake the salmon for 15-20 minutes, or until well done.

6. Serve with a side of steamed asparagus or roasted veggies.

Prep Time: 25 minutes

Servings: 4

5. Quinoa and Black Bean Stuffed Peppers

Ingredients:

- Cut 4 bell peppers in half and remove seeds

- Cook 1 cup of quinoa

- One can (15 oz) of black beans, drained and rinsed

- 1 cup corn kernels, fresh or frozen

- Add 1 cup chopped tomatoes

- 1 teaspoon cumin

- 1 teaspoon of chili powder

- Add Salt and pepper to taste

Preparation:

1. Preheat your oven to 375°F (190°C).

2. In a bowl, add the cooked quinoa, black beans, corn, chopped tomatoes, cumin, chili powder, salt, and pepper.

3. Fill each bell pepper half with quinoa mixture.

4. Transfer the filled peppers to a baking sheet.

5. Bake for 20 to 25 minutes, or until the peppers are soft.

6. Just before serving, garnish with chopped cilantro.

Prep Time: 40 minutes

Servings: 8 halves

6. Cauliflower Rice Bowls with Vegetables

Ingredients:

- 1 grated head cauliflower (to resemble rice)

- 2 tablespoons of olive oil

- 1 finely chopped onion,

- 2 shredded carrots,

- 1 diced zucchini,

- 1 cup of broccoli florets

- 2 tablespoons of low-sodium soy sauce

- 1 teaspoon of sesame oil

- Sesame seeds as garnish

Preparation:

1. Pulse cauliflower in a food processor until it looks like rice.

2. Increase the olive oil temperature in a large pan over medium heat.

3. Sauté the chopped onion until transparent, then add the shredded carrots, diced zucchini, and broccoli florets.

4. Stir cauliflower rice into the skillet until combined.

5. Drizzle soy sauce and sesame oil over the mixture and stir well.

6. Cook for another 5-7 minutes until the veggies are cooked.

7. Just before serving, garnish with sesame seeds.

Prep Time: 30 minutes

Servings: 4

7. Egg White Vegetable Omelet

Ingredients:

- 4 white eggs

- 1/2 cup of sliced bell peppers,

- 1/2 cup of chopped spinach,

- 1/4 cup of chopped tomatoes,

- One tablespoon of olive oil

- Add Salt and pepper to taste

Preparation:

1. In a mixing basin, combine the egg whites and whisk until foamy.

2. Heat olive oil in a nonstick pan over medium heat.

3. Add the bell peppers, spinach, and tomatoes to the pan and sauté until soft.

4. Spread the egg whites over the veggies equally.

5. Cook until the edges are firm, then fold the omelet in half.

6. Season with salt and pepper, then heat until the omelet is fully cooked.

Prep Time: 15 minutes

Servings: 1

8. Berry Smoothie Bowl

Ingredients:

- 1 cup of mixed berries like strawberries, blueberries, and raspberries

- 1/2 sliced banana,

- 1/2 cup of Greek yogurt

- 1/4 cup of granola

- One tablespoon of honey

Preparation:

1. Blend berries and banana until smooth.

2. Transfer the berry mixture to a basin.

3. Add Greek yogurt, oats, and a sprinkle of honey.

Prep Time: 10 minutes

Servings: 1

9. Shrimp and Vegetable Skewers

Ingredients:

- 12 big peeled and deveined shrimp

- 1 sliced zucchini,

- 1 diced bell pepper,

- 1 chopped red onion,

- Two tablespoons of olive oil

- 1 teaspoon of dried oregano

- 1 teaspoon of garlic powder

- Lemon wedges to serve

Preparation:

1. Preheat your grill or grill pan.

2. In a mixing dish, combine shrimp, zucchini, bell pepper, and red onion with olive oil, oregano, and garlic powder.

3. Thread shrimp and veggies on skewers.

4. Grill for 3-4 minutes on each side, or until the shrimp are opaque.

5. Serve with lemon wedges.

Prep Time: 20 minutes

Servings: 2

10. Turkey and Vegetable Stir-Fry

Ingredients:

- 1 pound of ground turkey

- 1 tablespoon of olive oil

- 1 sliced bell pepper,

- 1 cup of trimmed snap peas,

- 1 julienned carrot,

- 2 tablespoons of low-sodium soy sauce

- 1 teaspoon of ground ginger

- 1 teaspoon of garlic powder

Preparation:

1. Brown the ground turkey in a pan over medium heat until fully done.

2. Remove any extra fat and keep it aside.

3. Heat olive oil in the same skillet, then add the bell pepper, snap peas, and carrot. Stir fry until the veggies are soft and crunchy.

4. Place the cooked turkey back in the skillet.

5. In a small bowl, combine the soy sauce, ground ginger, and garlic powder. Pour over the turkey and veggies, stirring well.

6. Cook for a further 5 minutes, making sure all of the ingredients are covered in the sauce.

Prep Time: 30 minutes

Servings: 4

11. Sweet Potato and Black Bean Salad

Ingredients:

- 2 diced sweet potatoes,

- 1 can (15 oz) black beans (drained and washed)

- 1 cup of halved cherry tomatoes,

- 1/4 cup of finely chopped red onion,

- 2 tablespoons of olive oil

- 1 tablespoon of balsamic vinegar

- Add Salt and pepper to taste

Preparation:

1. Steam or boil sweet potato cubes until soft. Allow them to cool.

2. In a large mixing basin, add sweet potatoes, black beans, cherry tomatoes, and red onions.

3. In a small bowl, combine olive oil, balsamic vinegar, salt, and pepper.

4. Pour the dressing over the salad and gently toss to mix.

5. Refrigerate for at least 30 minutes before to serving.

Prep Time: 40 minutes

Servings: 4

12. Spinach and Strawberry Salad with Almonds

Ingredients:

- 4 cups of fresh spinach leaves

- 1 cup of sliced strawberries,

- 1/4 cup of sliced almonds,

- Two tablespoons of balsamic vinaigrette

- 1 tablespoon of feta cheese (optional)

Preparation:

1. To prepare, mix together fresh spinach, cut strawberries, and almonds in a big bowl.

2. Drizzle the salad with balsamic vinaigrette and gently toss to coat.

3. Optional: top with crumbled feta cheese.

4. Serve immediately.

Prep Time: 15 minutes

Servings: 4

13. Lemon Garlic Roasted Chicken Thighs

Ingredients:

- 4, bone-in, skin-on chicken thighs

- 2 tablespoons of olive oil

- 2 chopped garlic cloves

- 1 lemon (juiced and zested)

- 1 teaspoon of dry rosemary

- Add Salt and pepper to taste

Preparation:

1. Preheat oven to 400°F (200°C).

2. In a mixing bowl, combine olive oil, minced garlic, lemon juice, lemon zest, dried rosemary, salt, and pepper.

3. Place the chicken thighs on a baking sheet, then brush with the mixture.

4. Roast the chicken in the oven for 25-30 minutes, or until golden brown and fully done.

5. Serve alongside steaming green beans or a side salad.

Prep Time: 40 minutes

Servings: 4

14. Cauliflower and Broccoli Soup

Ingredients:

- 1 chopped head of cauliflower

- 2 cups of broccoli florets

- Chop one onion

- cut two garlic cloves

- Add 4 cups of low-sodium vegetable broth and 1 teaspoon of dried thyme

- Add Salt and pepper to taste

Preparation:

1. Cook chopped onion and garlic in a large saucepan until softened.

2. Combine the cauliflower, broccoli, vegetable broth, dried thyme, salt, and pepper.

3. Bring to a boil, then decrease the heat and simmer for 20-25 minutes, or until the veggies are cooked.

4. Using an immersion blender or a conventional blender, mix the soup until it is smooth.

5. Adjust the spice as needed and serve hot.

Prep Time: 35 minutes

Servings: 6

15. Turkey and Vegetable Casserole

Ingredients:

- 1 pound of ground turkey

- 1 cup of cooked brown rice

- 1 , sliced zucchini

- 1 sliced yellow squash,

- 1 chopped bell pepper,

- One cup of tomato sauce

- One teaspoon of dried oregano

- To prepare, add 1 teaspoon dried basil, salt and pepper to taste

- 1 cup of shredded low-fat mozzarella cheese

Preparation:

1. Preheat oven to 375°F (190°C).

2. Brown ground turkey in a pan until heated through. Drain any extra fat.

3. In a large mixing bowl, add the cooked turkey, brown rice, zucchini, yellow squash, bell pepper, tomato sauce, dried oregano, basil, salt, and pepper.

4. Place the mixture in a baking dish and top with shredded mozzarella cheese.

5. Bake for 20-25 minutes, or until the cheese melts and bubbles.

6. Let it cool somewhat before serving.

Prep Time: 45 minutes

Servings: 6

16. Lemon Herb Tilapia

Ingredients:

- 4 tilapia fillets

- 2 tablespoons of olive oil

- 1 sliced lemon,

- 1 teaspoon of dried parsley

- 1 teaspoon of dried dill

- Salt and pepper to taste

Preparation:

1. Preheat oven to 375°F (190°C).

2. Lay the tilapia fillets on a baking sheet.

3. Drizzle olive oil over the fillets and sprinkle with dried parsley, dill, salt, and pepper.

4. Garnish each fillet with lemon wedges.

5. Bake for 15 to 18 minutes, or until the tilapia is cooked through.

6. Serve with a bowl of quinoa or steamed asparagus.

Prep Time: 25 minutes

Servings: 4

17. Mediterranean Chickpea Salad

Ingredients:

- 2 cans (15 oz each) of drained and rinsed chickpeas

- 1 diced cucumber,

- 1 halved cup cherry tomatoes,

- 1/2 finely chopped red onion,

- 1/4 cup of crumbled feta cheese,

- 2 tablespoons of olive oil

- 1 tablespoon of red wine vinegar

- 1 teaspoon of dried oregano

- Add Salt and pepper to taste

Preparation:

Mix chickpeas, cucumber, cherry tomatoes, red onion, and feta cheese in a big bowl.

2. In a small dish, combine the olive oil, red wine vinegar, dried oregano, salt, and pepper.

3. Pour the dressing over the salad and gently toss to mix.

4. Refrigerate for a minimum of 30 minutes before serving.

Prep Time: 20 minutes

Servings: 6

18. Roasted Vegetable and Quinoa Bowl

Ingredients:

- 1 cup of cooked quinoa

- 1 sliced zucchini,

- 1 sliced red bell pepper,

- 1 sliced yellow bell pepper,

- One cup of cherry tomatoes

- Add 2 tablespoons of olive oil

- 1 teaspoon of dried thyme

- Add Salt and pepper to taste

Preparation:

1. Preheat your oven to 400°F (200°C).

2. In a mixing dish, combine zucchini, red bell pepper, yellow bell pepper, and cherry tomatoes with olive oil, dried thyme, salt, and pepper.

3. Set up the veggies on a baking sheet.

4. Roast in the oven for 20-25 minutes, or until the veggies are soft and faintly browned.

5. Place the roasted veggies over a bed of cooked quinoa.

Prep Time: 30 minutes

Servings: 4

19. Turkey and Vegetable Quinoa Bowl

Ingredients:

- 1 cup of cooked quinoa,

- 1 pound of ground turkey

- 1 tablespoon of olive oil

- Dice one bell pepper and one zucchini

- Halve one cup of cherry tomatoes

- Mince two cloves of garlic

- One teaspoon of dried Italian herbs

- Add Salt and pepper to taste

Preparation:

1. To prepare, sauté ground turkey in olive oil in a pan until cooked through. Drain any extra fat.

2. In the skillet, combine diced bell pepper, zucchini, cherry tomatoes, minced garlic, dried Italian herbs, salt, and pepper.

3. Cook for another 5-7 minutes, until the veggies are soft.

4. Arrange the turkey and veggie combination on a bed of cooked quinoa.

Prep Time: 30 minutes

Servings: 4

20. Broccoli and Chicken Stir-Fry

Ingredients:

- 1 pound of boneless and skinless chicken breasts, sliced

- Two cups of broccoli florets

- One red bell pepper, cut

- 1 cup snap peas, trimmed

- Two tablespoons of low-sodium soy sauce

- To prepare, combine 1 tablespoon sesame oil, 1 teaspoon grated ginger, and 2 chopped garlic cloves

- One tablespoon of olive oil

Preparation:

1. Increase the olive oil temperature in a large pan over medium-high heat.

2. Add the sliced chicken and sauté until browned and cooked through.

3. Take out the chicken from the pan and set it aside.

4. In the same pan, combine the broccoli, red bell pepper, and snap peas. Sauté the veggies for 5-7 minutes, or until soft and crisp.

5. Return the cooked chicken to the skillet.

6. In a small bowl, combine soy sauce, sesame oil, grated ginger, and chopped garlic. Pour over the chicken and veggies and mix to incorporate.

7. Cook for a further 3-4 minutes, or until everything is well covered with the sauce.

Prep Time: 25 minutes

Servings: 4

CONCLUSION

In closing this CKD Stage 4 diet cookbook for seniors, I underline the transforming effect of mindful eating on kidney health.

Each dish embodies a dedication to flavor, nutrition, and kidney-friendly ingredients, resulting in a delectable journey to wellness.

As we conclude our gastronomic adventure, remember that these meals are more than simply recipes; they are a testament to nurturing your kidneys with each mouthful.

Embrace this comprehensive approach and enjoy the path to optimal health. Let the colorful tastes and kidney-friendly options be a celebration of life, providing both food and joy.

May this cookbook inspire a greater awareness for the link between culinary enjoyment and renal heath as you embark on your journey to a flourishing and energetic retirement.

As we say goodbye, I want to express my deepest appreciation for reading the pages of our CKD Stage 4 diet cookbook for seniors.

Your road to kidney health is a collaborative effort, and I appreciate your faith in these recipes. May each meal offer both sustenance and delight to your table.

Remember, this cookbook is a tool to help you achieve your health goals, and your commitment to making kidney-friendly choices is admirable.

Thank you for letting this culinary journey become part of your story. I wish you good health, happiness, and delicious moments ahead.

With appreciation,

Patricia Camire

HAPPY COOKING!